# OPTAVIA DIET COOKBOOK FOR BEGINNERS

*THE BEGINNER'S OPTAVIA DIET GUIDE TO ACHIEVE A RAPID WEIGHT LOSS WITHOUT OVERTHINKING ABOUT MEAL PLANNING*

(Harold Williams)

1

# CONTENTS

# What Is the Optavia Diet?

The Optavia Diet provides convenience to people as it is a convenient meal replacement that removes the guesswork for many of its dieters. The Optavia Diet, previously known as Medifast, was developed by Dr. William Vitale and encourages people to eat healthy in order to achieve sustainable weight loss.

Under this diet regimen, dieters follow a weight plan including five fuelings a day as well as one lean green meal a day. One of the popular diet plans that Optavia has to offer is the 5&1 plan that is designed for rapid weight loss. With this diet plan, users need to eat five of Optavia's fuelings and one lean and green meal daily.

With the meal replacement and lean green meals, this diet is perfect for people who do not only want to lose weight but also for people who want to transition from their old unhealthy habits to a healthier one. Thus, this is perfect for people who suffer from gout, diabetes, as well as people who are in their senior years.

Because it is a commercial diet, it has been subjected to different studies involving its efficacy. Studies have noted that people can lose weight in as little as 8 weeks therefore this is one of the most efficient diet regimens there is that people can adapt and eventually embrace as part of their lifestyles. Read on to learn about the Optavia Diet.
What To Eat

Depending on the type of diet plan that you choose, you have to eat a number of lean and green meals that are comprised mainly of lean proteins and non-starchy vegetables. Although this diet regimen is not as restrictive as other diet regimens, this means that there are plenty of foods that are compliant to this diet including healthy fats. Thus, below are the types of foods that you can eat while following the Optavia Diet.

**Optavia fuelings:** The Optavia Diet is famous for its Optavia fuelings that involve pre-packaged foods that dieters can eat. There are more than 60 soups, shakes, bars, and other fueling products that you can consume as your meal replacements.

**Lean meats:** Lean and green meals require you to make foods out of lean meats. There are three categories of lean meats identified by Optavia including (1) lean, (2) leaner, and (3) leanest. Lean meats include salmon, pork chops, and lamb while leaner meats include chicken breasts and swordfish. Leanest meats include egg whites, shrimp, and cod.

**Green and non-starchy vegetables:** Non-starchy vegetables are further identified into (1) lower carb, (2) moderate carb, and (3) higher carb. Lower carbs include all types of salad greens and green leafy vegetables. Moderate carb vegetables include summer squash and cauliflower. Lastly, high carb vegetables include peppers and broccoli.

**Healthy fats:** Healthy fats are encouraged for people who follow the Optavia Diet. These include healthy fats such as olive oil, walnut oil, flaxseed, and avocado. However, it is important to consume two servings of healthy fats to still keep up with the Optavia Diet.

**Others:** Once dieters are able to achieve their weight loss goals through meal replacements, they can start consuming other foods to maintain their ideal weight. These include low-fat dairy, fresh fruits, and whole grains. You can also consume meatless alternatives including 2 cups egg substitute, and 5 ounces seitan. For low-fat dairy, you are allowed to consume 1 ½ cups 1% cottage cheese and 12 ounces of non-fat Greek yogurt.

# What Not to Eat

Similar to other diet regimens, the Optavia Diet also discourages dieters not to eat certain types of foods. This section will discuss the foods that are non-compliant to the principles of the Optavia Diet.

**Indulgent desserts:** This diet regimen discourages the consumption of indulgent desserts such as cakes, ice cream, cookies, and all kinds of pastries. While eating these foods is discouraged during the first few weeks of following the diet, moderate consumption of sweet treats such as fresh fruits and yogurts can be integrated into one's diet.

**Sugary beverages:** Similar to indulgent desserts, sugary beverages are also discouraged among those who follow the Optavia Diet. These include soda, fruit juices, and energy drinks.

**Unhealthy fats:** Fats such as butter, shortening, and commercial salad dressings contain large amounts of calories that are not good for people who are trying to lose weight. Moreover, they also contain preservatives and salt that is not good for the overall health.

**Alcohol:** Those who follow the Optavia Diet should limit their alcohol intake to 5 ounces of alcohol daily.

# The Benefits of The Optavia Diet

The Optavia Diet has a high success rate especially among people who want to lose weight. But more than losing weight, there are so many benefits of following the Optavia Diet. Below are the many benefits that people can enjoy when following this particular diet.

**Better for portion control:** Perhaps one of the most challenging facets of dieting is portion control. Many people find it difficult to control the amount of food while dieting but the Optavia Diet is really strict when it comes to its fueling phase as it strictly implements portion control thanks to its pre-packaged fueling foods.

**Structured eating plan:** The Optavia Diet follows a structured eating plan thus making it very easy to follow. Everything is indicated on their website so you do not need to figure everything else on your own.

**Builds a healthy relationship with food:** The problem with most people why they revert to their old eating habits is that they do not have a good relationship with food. But with the Optavia Diet, it is backed by a solid and supportive community that helps each other out. With the support of great people, it is easier for people to develop healthy eating habits as they gain appreciation for the many options and support that they have.

**Better overall health:** The Optavia Diet was not only designed only for weight loss. In fact, it was also designed for people to achieve better overall health. Several studies have noted that this diet is also associated with lowering blood and sugar levels due to its limited Sodium intake.

# How to Start the Optavia Diet?

The Optavia Diet has two unique phases: Initial and Maintenance Phases. Upon enrollment, you will be assigned a diet coach that will help you undertake all the necessary things in order to be a successful dieter. So, if you are wondering what are the steps that you need to undertake while following the two phases, then this section will discuss just that.

The initial phase is when people are encouraged to limit their calorie intake from 800 to 1,000 calories for the next 12 weeks or until the dieter loses 12 pounds. For this phase, dieters are encouraged to consume lean and green meals five to seven times daily. Moreover, dieters are also encouraged to consume 1 optional snack including sugar-free gelatin, celery sticks, and 12 ounces of nuts.

The maintenance phase, on the other hand, is implemented once you have already lost the 12 pounds from your initial weight. During this phase, you can increase your calorie intake to 1,550 daily. This phase can last for 6 weeks. Moreover, you are also allowed to incorporate other foods such as whole grains, fruits, and low-fat dairy into your diet.

After the maintenance phase, you are not ready to follow your specific Optavia Diet plan. This is also the time when you need to consume not only lean and green meals but also fueling foods. The number of meals depends on the specific diet plan you choose. For instance, if you opt for the 3&3 Optavia plan, you need to consume three lean and green meals and three fuelings.

# How to Follow the Optavia Diet?

While the Optavia Diet is all about delivering weight loss to its dieters, the success of dieters still largely depends on how they approach this particular diet regimen. Thus, if you want to become successful, below are the tips that you should do while following the Optavia Diet.

Opt for foods that are cooked using healthy cooking methods. Healthy cooking methods include baking, grilling, poaching, and broiling. Avoid frying your foods as cooking oil increases the calorie content of your food.

Portion sizes of your food should follow the Optavia recommendations. This means that the portion sizes refer to the cooked weight and not the raw weight of the ingredients that you are using.

Opt for foods that are rich in Omega-3 fatty acids such as tuna salmon, mackerel, trout, herring, and many other cold-water fishes. Omega-3 fatty acids contribute to lowering inflammation in the body.

Choose meatless alternatives such as tofu and tempeh. They rich in proteins but not too much on calories.

Following the program at all costs even if you are dining out. This means that you have to consume healthy meals when you eat out and make sure that you stay away from alcohol.

# Following the Optavia Diet

The developers of the Optavia Diet strives to be transparent when it comes to developing their many regimens and plans. But if you have questions about this diet regimen, then below are some FAQs that many people ask.

## Which Optavia Diet plan is good for me?

As there are so many diet plans offered by Optavia, it is important to get in touch with a certified Optavia coach to learn about the many options that you have. It is crucial that you do not second guess the diet plan that you are going to follow as each diet plan is designed to fit a particular profile. For instance, if you are a very active person, you can take on the Optavia 5&1 plan. But then, the coach will also look at other factors such as your age and health risks so that you can be matched with the right Optavia Diet Plan.

## Can I skip the fuelings?

No. You must stick with fuelings if you want to successfully follow the Optavia Diet. Fuelings are designed to provide the body with balanced amounts of macronutrients that can promote an efficient fat-burning state to help people lose fat without losing energy. The problem if you skip fueling is that you may miss out on important nutrients that might lead to fatigue while following this diet. The body feels fatigued because it cannot compensate for the lack of nutrients while being calorie deficient.

## Can I rearrange my fuelings?

Yes. If you are a busy person with a dynamic schedule, then you can rearrange the timing on when you will take your fueling meals. The Optavia Diet is not strict about rearranging meals as long as you consume your meals within 24 hours. This versatility on your eating schedule makes it perfect for people who also have unusual schedules including those who work at night or beyond regular working hours. So how do you time your fuelings? Just make sure that you eat your meals every two or three hours throughout the time that you are awake. Your first meal should be taken an hour after waking up to ensure optimal blood sugar levels. This is also great for hunger control.

# LEAN & GREEN RECIPES

## Pesto Zucchini Noodles

**Time**: 30 minutes

**Serve:** 4

**Ingredients:**

- 4 zucchini, spiralized
- 1 tbsp avocado oil
- 2 garlic cloves, chopped
- 2/3 cup olive oil
- 1/3 cup parmesan cheese, grated
- 2 cups fresh basil
- 1/3 cup almonds
- 1/8 tsp black pepper
- ¾ tsp sea salt

**Directions:**

1. Add zucchini noodles into a colander and sprinkle with ¼ teaspoon of salt. Cover and let sit for 30 minutes. Drain zucchini noodles well and pat dry.
2. Preheat the oven to 400 F.
3. Place almonds on a parchment-lined baking sheet and bake for 6-8 minutes.
4. Transfer toasted almonds into the food processor and process until coarse.
5. Add olive oil, cheese, basil, garlic, pepper, and remaining salt in a food processor with almonds and process until pesto texture.
6. Heat avocado oil in a large pan over medium-high heat.
7. Add zucchini noodles and cook for 4-5 minutes.
8. Pour pesto over zucchini noodles, mix well and cook for 1 minute.
9. Serve immediately with baked salmon.

**Nutritional Value (Amount per Serving):**

Calories 525  Fat 47.4 g  Carbs 9.3 g  Sugar 3.8 g  Protein 16.6 g  Cholesterol 30 mg

# Baked Cod & Vegetables

**Time:** 30 minutes

**Serve:** 4

**Ingredients:**

- 1 lb cod fillets
- 8 oz asparagus, chopped
- 3 cups broccoli, chopped
- ¼ cup parsley, minced
- ½ tsp lemon pepper seasoning
- ½ tsp paprika
- ¼ cup olive oil
- ¼ cup lemon juice
- 1 tsp salt

**Directions:**

1. Preheat the oven to 400 F. Line baking sheet with parchment paper and set aside.
2. In a small bowl, mix together lemon juice, paprika, olive oil, lemon pepper seasoning, and salt.
3. Place fish fillets in the middle of the parchment paper. Place broccoli and asparagus around the fish fillets.
4. Pour lemon juice mixture over the fish fillets and top with parsley.
5. Bake in preheated oven for 13-15 minutes.
6. Serve and enjoy.

**Nutritional Value (Amount per Serving):**

Calories 240  Fat 14.1 g  Carbs 7.6 g  Sugar 2.6 g  Protein 23.7 g  Cholesterol 56 mg

# Parmesan Zucchini

**Time:** 30 minutes

**Serve**: 4

**Ingredients:**

- 4 zucchini, quartered lengthwise
- 2 tbsp fresh parsley, chopped
- 2 tbsp olive oil
- ¼ tsp garlic powder
- ½ tsp dried basil
- ½ tsp dried oregano
- ½ tsp dried thyme
- ½ cup parmesan cheese, grated
- Pepper
- Salt

**Directions:**

1. Preheat the oven to 350 F. Line baking sheet with parchment paper and set aside.
2. In a small bowl, mix together parmesan cheese, garlic powder, basil, oregano, thyme, pepper, and salt.
3. Arrange zucchini onto the prepared baking sheet and drizzle with oil and sprinkle with parmesan cheese mixture.
4. Bake in preheated oven for 15 minutes then broil for 2 minutes or until lightly golden brown.
5. Garnish with parsley and serve immediately.

**Nutritional Value (Amount per Serving):**

Calories 244  Fat 16.4 g  Carbs 7 g  Sugar 3.5 g  Protein 14.5 g  Cholesterol 30 mg

# Chicken Zucchini Noodles

**Time:** 25 minutes

**Serve:** 2

**Ingredients:**

- 1 large zucchini, spiralized
- 1 chicken breast, skinless & boneless
- ½ tbsp jalapeno, minced
- 2 garlic cloves, minced
- ½ tsp ginger, minced
- ½ tbsp fish sauce
- 2 tbsp coconut cream
- ½ tbsp honey
- ½ lime juice
- 1 tbsp peanut butter
- 1 carrot, chopped
- 2 tbsp cashews, chopped
- ¼ cup fresh cilantro, chopped
- 1 tbsp olive oil
- Pepper
- Salt

**Directions:**

1. Heat olive oil in a pan over medium-high heat.
2. Season chicken breast with pepper and salt. Once the oil is hot then add chicken breast into the pan and cook for 3-4 minutes per side or until cooked.
3. Remove chicken breast from pan. Shred chicken breast with a fork and set aside.
4. In a small bowl, mix together peanut butter, jalapeno, garlic, ginger, fish sauce, coconut cream, honey, and lime juice. Set aside.
5. In a large mixing bowl, combine together spiralized zucchini, carrots, cashews, cilantro, and shredded chicken.
6. Pour peanut butter mixture over zucchini noodles and toss to combine.
7. Serve immediately and enjoy.

**Nutritional Value (Amount per Serving):**

Calories 353  Fat 21.1 g  Carbs 20.5 g  Sugar 10.8 g  Protein 24.5 g  Cholesterol 54 mg

# Tomato Cucumber Avocado Salad

**Time:** 15 minutes

**Serve:** 4

**Ingredients:**

- 12 oz cherry tomatoes, cut in half
- 5 small cucumbers, chopped
- 3 small avocados, chopped
- ½ tsp ground black pepper
- 2 tbsp olive oil
- 2 tbsp fresh lemon juice
- ¼ cup fresh cilantro, chopped
- 1 tsp sea salt

**Directions:**

1. Add cherry tomatoes, cucumbers, avocados, and cilantro into the large mixing bowl and mix well.
2. Mix together olive oil, lemon juice, black pepper, and salt and pour over salad.
3. Toss well and serve immediately.

**Nutritional Value (Amount per Serving):**

Calories 442  Fat 37.1 g  Carbs 30.3 g  Sugar 9.4 g  Protein 6.2 g  Cholesterol 0 mg

# Creamy Cauliflower Soup

**Time:** 30 minutes

**Serve:** 6

**Ingredients:**

- 5 cups cauliflower rice
- 8 oz cheddar cheese, grated
- 2 cups unsweetened almond milk
- 2 cups vegetable stock
- 2 tbsp water
- 1 small onion, chopped
- 2 garlic cloves, minced
- 1 tbsp olive oil
- Pepper
- Salt

**Directions:**

1. Heat olive oil in a large stockpot over medium heat.
2. Add onion and garlic and cook for 1-2 minutes.
3. Add cauliflower rice and water. Cover and cook for 5-7 minutes.
4. Now add vegetable stock and almond milk and stir well. Bring to boil.
5. Turn heat to low and simmer for 5 minutes.
6. Turn off the heat. Slowly add cheddar cheese and stir until smooth.
7. Season soup with pepper and salt.
8. Stir well and serve hot.

**Nutritional Value (Amount per Serving):**

Calories 214  Fat 16.5 g  Carbs 7.3 g  Sugar 3 g  Protein 11.6 g  Cholesterol 40 mg

# Taco Zucchini Boats

**Time:** 70 minutes

**Serve:** 4

**Ingredients:**

- 4 medium zucchinis, cut in half lengthwise
- ¼ cup fresh cilantro, chopped
- ½ cup cheddar cheese, shredded
- ¼ cup water
- 4 oz tomato sauce
- 2 tbsp bell pepper, mined
- ½ small onion, minced
- ½ tsp oregano
- 1 tsp paprika
- 1 tsp chili powder
- 1 tsp cumin
- 1 tsp garlic powder
- 1 lb lean ground turkey
- ½ cup salsa
- 1 tsp kosher salt

**Directions:**

1. Preheat the oven to 400 F.
2. Add ¼ cup of salsa in the bottom of the baking dish.
3. Using a spoon hollow out the center of the zucchini halves.
4. Chop the scooped-out flesh of zucchini and set aside ¾ of a cup chopped flesh.
5. Add zucchini halves in the boiling water and cook for 1 minute. Remove zucchini halves from water.
6. Add ground turkey in a large pan and cook until meat is no longer pink. Add spices and mix well.
7. Add reserved zucchini flesh, water, tomato sauce, bell pepper, and onion. Stir well and cover, simmer over low heat for 20 minutes.

8. Stuff zucchini boats with taco meat and top each with one tablespoon of shredded cheddar cheese.
9. Place zucchini boats in baking dish. Cover dish with foil and bake in preheated oven for 35 minutes.
10. Top with remaining salsa and chopped cilantro.
11. Serve and enjoy.

**Nutritional Value (Amount per Serving):**

Calories 297  Fat 13.7 g  Carbs 17.2 g  Sugar 9.3 g  Protein 30.2 g  Cholesterol 96 mg

# Healthy Broccoli Salad

**Time:** 25 minutes

**Serve:** 6

**Ingredients:**

- 3 cups broccoli, chopped
- 1 tbsp apple cider vinegar
- ½ cup Greek yogurt
- 2 tbsp sunflower seeds
- 3 bacon slices, cooked and chopped
- 1/3 cup onion, sliced
- ¼ tsp stevia

**Directions:**

1. In a mixing bowl, mix together broccoli, onion, and bacon.
2. In a small bowl, mix together yogurt, vinegar, and stevia and pour over broccoli mixture. Stir to combine.
3. Sprinkle sunflower seeds on top of the salad.
4. Store salad in the refrigerator for 30 minutes.
5. Serve and enjoy.

**Nutritional Value (Amount per Serving):**

Calories 90  Fat 4.9 g  Carbs 5.4 g  Sugar 2.5 g  Protein 6.2 g  Cholesterol 12 mg

# Delicious Zucchini Quiche

**Time:** 60 minutes

**Serve:** 8

**Ingredients:**

- 6 eggs
- 2 medium zucchini, shredded
- ½ tsp dried basil
- 2 garlic cloves, minced
- 1 tbsp dry onion, minced
- 2 tbsp parmesan cheese, grated
- 2 tbsp fresh parsley, chopped
- ½ cup olive oil
- 1 cup cheddar cheese, shredded
- ¼ cup coconut flour
- ¾ cup almond flour
- ½ tsp salt

**Directions:**

1. Preheat the oven to 350 F. Grease 9-inch pie dish and set aside.
2. Squeeze out excess liquid from zucchini.
3. Add all ingredients into the large bowl and mix until well combined. Pour into the prepared pie dish.
4. Bake in preheated oven for 45-60 minutes or until set.
5. Remove from the oven and let it cool completely.
6. Slice and serve.

**Nutritional Value (Amount per Serving):**

Calories 288  Fat 26.3 g  Carbs 5 g  Sugar 1.6 g  Protein 11 g  Cholesterol 139 mg

# Turkey Spinach Egg Muffins

**Time:** 30 minutes

**Serve:** 3

**Ingredients:**

- 5 egg whites
- 2 eggs
- ¼ cup cheddar cheese, shredded
- ¼ cup spinach, chopped
- ¼ cup milk
- 3 lean breakfast turkey sausage
- Pepper
- Salt

**Directions:**

1. Preheat the oven to 350 F. Grease muffin tray cups and set aside.
2. In a pan, brown the turkey sausage links over medium-high heat until sausage is brown from all the sides.
3. Cut sausage in ½-inch pieces and set aside.
4. In a large bowl, whisk together eggs, egg whites, milk, pepper, and salt. Stir in spinach.
5. Pour egg mixture into the prepared muffin tray.
6. Divide sausage and cheese evenly between each muffin cup.
7. Bake in preheated oven for 20 minutes or until muffins are set.
8. Serve warm and enjoy.

**Nutritional Value (Amount per Serving):**

Calories 123  Fat 6.8 g  Carbs 1.9 g  Sugar 1.6 g  Protein 13.3 g  Cholesterol 123 mg

# Chicken Casserole

**Time:** 40 minutes

**Serve:** 4

**Ingredients:**

- 1 lb cooked chicken, shredded
- ¼ cup Greek yogurt
- 1 cup cheddar cheese, shredded
- ½ cup salsa
- 4 oz cream cheese, softened
- 4 cups cauliflower florets
- 1/8 tsp black pepper
- ½ tsp kosher salt

**Directions:**

1. Add cauliflower florets into the microwave-safe dish and cook for 10 minutes or until tender.
2. Add cream cheese and microwave for 30 seconds more. Stir well.
3. Add chicken, yogurt, cheddar cheese, salsa, pepper, and salt and stir everything well.
4. Preheat the oven to 375 F.
5. Bake in preheated oven for 20 minutes.
6. Serve hot and enjoy.

**Nutritional Value (Amount per Serving):**

Calories 429  Fat 23 g  Carbs 9.6 g  Sugar 4.7 g  Protein 45.4 g  Cholesterol 149 mg

# Shrimp Cucumber Salad

**Time:** 20 minutes

**Serve:** 4

**Ingredients:**

- 1 lb shrimp, cooked
- 1 bell pepper, sliced
- 2 green onions, sliced
- ½ cup fresh cilantro, chopped
- 2 cucumbers, sliced
- For dressing:
- 2 tbsp fresh mint leaves, chopped
- 1 tsp sesame seeds
- ½ tsp red pepper flakes
- 1 tbsp olive oil
- ¼ cup rice wine vinegar
- ¼ cup lime juice
- 1 Serrano chili pepper, minced
- 3 garlic cloves, minced
- ½ tsp salt

**Directions:**

1. In a small bowl, whisk together all dressing ingredients and set aside.
2. In a mixing bowl, mix together shrimp, bell pepper, green onion, cilantro, and cucumbers.
3. Pour dressing over salad and toss well.
4. Serve and enjoy.

**Nutritional Value (Amount per Serving):**

Calories 219  Fat 6.1 g  Carbs 11.3 g  Sugar 4.2 g  Protein 27.7 g  Cholesterol 239 mg

# Asparagus & Shrimp Stir Fry

**Time:** 20 minutes

**Serve:** 4

**Ingredients:**

- 1 lb asparagus
- 1 lb shrimp
- 2 tbsp lemon juice
- 1 tbsp soy sauce
- 1 tsp ginger, minced
- 1 garlic clove, minced
- 1 tsp red pepper flakes
- ¼ cup olive oil
- Pepper
- Salt

**Directions:**

1. Heat 2 tablespoons of oil in a large pan over medium-high heat.
2. Add shrimp to the pan and season with red pepper flakes, pepper, and salt and cook for 5 minutes.
3. Remove shrimp from pan and set aside.
4. Add remaining oil in the same pan. Add garlic, ginger, and asparagus and stir frequently and cook until asparagus is tender about 5 minutes.
5. Return shrimp to the pan. Add lemon juice and soy sauce and stir until well combined.
6. Serve hot and enjoy.

**Nutritional Value (Amount per Serving):**

Calories 274  Fat 14.8 g  Carbs 7.4 g  Sugar 2.4 g  Protein 28.8 g  Cholesterol 239 mg

# Turkey Burgers

**Time:** 30 minutes

**Serve:** 4

**Ingredients:**

- 1 lb lean ground turkey
- 2 green onions, sliced
- ¼ cup basil leaves, shredded
- 2 garlic cloves, minced
- 2 medium zucchini, shredded and squeeze out all the liquid
- ½ tsp black pepper
- ½ tsp sea salt

**Directions:**

1. Heat grill to medium heat.
2. Add all ingredients into the mixing bowl and mix until well combined.
3. Make four equal shapes of patties from the mixture.
4. Spray one piece of foil with cooking spray.
5. Place prepared patties on the foil and grill for 10 minutes. Turn patties to the other side and grill for 10 minutes more.
6. Serve and enjoy.

**Nutritional Value (Amount per Serving):**

Calories 183  Fat 8.3 g  Carbs 4.5 g  Sugar 1.9 g  Protein 23.8 g  Cholesterol 81 mg

# Broccoli Kale Salmon Burgers

**Time:** 30 minutes

**Serve:** 5

**Ingredients:**

- 2 eggs
- ½ cup onion, chopped
- ½ cup broccoli, chopped
- ½ cup kale, chopped
- ½ tsp garlic powder
- 2 tbsp lemon juice
- ½ cup almond flour
- 15 oz can salmon, drained and bones removed
- ½ tsp salt

**Directions:**

1. Line one plate with parchment paper and set aside.
2. Add all ingredients into the large bowl and mix until well combined.
3. Make five equal shapes of patties from mixture and place on a prepared plate.
4. Place plate in the refrigerator for 30 minutes.
5. Spray a large pan with cooking spray and heat over medium heat.
6. Once the pan is hot then add patties and cook for 5-7 minutes per side.
7. Serve and enjoy.

**Nutritional Value (Amount per Serving):**

Calories 221  Fat 12.6 g  Carbs 5.2 g  Sugar 1.4 g  Protein 22.1 g  Cholesterol 112 mg

# Pan Seared Cod

**Time:** 25 minutes

**Serve:** 4

**Ingredients:**

- 1 ¾ lbs cod fillets
- 1 tbsp ranch seasoning
- 4 tsp olive oil

**Directions:**

1. Heat oil in a large pan over medium-high heat.
2. Season fish fillets with ranch seasoning.
3. Once the oil is hot then place fish fillets in a pan and cook for 6-8 minutes on each side.
4. Serve immediately and enjoy.

**Nutritional Value (Amount per Serving):**

Calories 207  Fat 6.4 g  Carbs 0 g  Sugar 0 g  Protein 35.4 g  Cholesterol 97 mg

# Quick Lemon Pepper Salmon

**Time:** 18 minutes

**Serve:** 4

**Ingredients:**

- 1 ½ lbs salmon fillets
- ½ tsp ground black pepper
- 1 tsp dried oregano
- 2 garlic cloves, minced
- ¼ cup olive oil
- 1 lemon juice
- 1 tsp sea salt

**Directions:**

1. In a large bowl, mix together lemon juice, olive oil, garlic, oregano, black pepper, and salt.
2. Add fish fillets in bowl and coat well with marinade and place in the refrigerator for 15 minutes.
3. Preheat the grill.
4. Brush grill grates with oil.
5. Place marinated salmon fillets on hot grill and cook for 4 minutes then turn salmon fillets to the other side and cook for 4 minutes more.
6. Serve and enjoy.

**Nutritional Value (Amount per Serving):**

Calories 340  Fat 23.3 g  Carbs 1.2 g  Sugar 0.3 g  Protein 33.3 g  Cholesterol 75 mg

# Healthy Salmon Salad

**Time:** 20 minutes

**Serve:** 2

**Ingredients:**

- 2 salmon fillets
- 2 tbsp olive oil
- ¼ cup onion, chopped
- 1 cucumber, peeled and sliced
- 1 avocado, diced
- 2 tomatoes, chopped
- 4 cups baby spinach
- Pepper
- Salt

**Directions:**

1. Heat oil in a pan over medium-high heat.
2. Season salmon fillets with pepper and salt. Place fish fillets in a pan and cook for 4-5 minutes.
3. Turn fish fillets and cook for 2-3 minutes more.
4. Divide remaining ingredients evenly between two bowls, then top with cooked fish fillet.
5. Serve and enjoy.

**Nutritional Value (Amount per Serving):**

Calories 350  Fat 23.2 g  Carbs 15.3 g  Sugar 6.6 g  Protein 25 g  Cholesterol 18 mg

# Pan Seared Tilapia

**Time:** 18 minutes

**Serve:** 2

**Ingredients:**

- 18 oz tilapia fillets
- ¼ tsp lemon pepper
- ½ tsp parsley flakes
- ¼ tsp garlic powder
- 1 tsp Cajun seasoning
- ½ tsp dried oregano
- 2 tbsp olive oil

**Directions:**

1. Heat olive oil in a pan over medium heat.
2. Season fish fillets with lemon pepper, parsley flakes, garlic powder, Cajun seasoning, and oregano.
3. Place fish fillets in the pan and cook for 3-4 minutes on each side.
4. Serve and enjoy.

**Nutritional Value (Amount per Serving):**

Calories 333  Fat 16.4 g  Carbs 0.7 g  Sugar 0.1 g  Protein 47.6 g  Cholesterol 124 mg

# Creamy Broccoli Soup

**Time:** 35 minutes

**Serve:** 8

**Ingredients:**

- 20 oz frozen broccoli, thawed and chopped
- ¼ tsp nutmeg
- 4 cups vegetable broth
- 1 potato, peeled and chopped
- 2 garlic cloves, peeled and chopped
- 1 large onion, chopped
- 1 tbsp olive oil
- Pepper
- Salt

**Directions:**

1. Heat oil in a large saucepan over medium heat.
2. Add garlic and onion and sauté until onion is tender.
3. Add potato, broccoli, and broth and bring to boil. Turn heat to low and simmer for 15 minutes or until vegetables are tender.
4. Using blender puree the soup until smooth. Season soup with nutmeg, pepper, and salt.
5. Serve and enjoy.

**Nutritional Value (Amount per Serving):**

Calories 84  Fat 2.7 g  Carbs 10.9 g  Sugar 2.6 g  Protein 5.1 g  Cholesterol 0 mg

# Tuna Muffins

**Time:** 35 minutes

**Serve:** 8

**Ingredients:**

- 2 eggs, lightly beaten
- 1 can tuna, flaked
- 1 tsp cayenne pepper
- 1/4 cup mayonnaise
- 1 celery stalk, chopped
- 1 1/2 cups cheddar cheese, shredded
- 1/4 cup sour cream
- Pepper
- Salt

**Directions:**

1. Preheat the oven to 350 F. Grease muffin tin and set aside.
2. Add all ingredients into the large bowl and mix until well combined and pour into the prepared muffin tin.
3. Bake for 25 minutes.
4. Serve and enjoy.

**Nutritional Value (Amount per Serving):**

Calories 185  Fat 14 g  Carbs 2.6 g  Sugar 0.7 g  Protein 13 g  Cholesterol 75 mg

# Chicken Cauliflower Rice

**Time:** 25 minutes

**Serve:** 4

**Ingredients:**

- 1 cauliflower head, chopped
- 2 cups cooked chicken, shredded
- 1 tsp olive oil
- 1 tsp garlic powder
- 1 tsp chili powder
- 1 tsp cumin
- 1/4 cup tomatoes, diced
- Salt

**Directions:**

1. Add cauliflower into the food processor and process until get rice size pieces.
2. Heat oil in a pan over high heat.
3. Add cauliflower rice and chicken in a pan and cook for 5-7 minutes.
4. Add garlic powder, chili powder, cumin, tomatoes, and salt. Stir well and cook for 7-10 minutes more.
5. Serve and enjoy.

**Nutritional Value (Amount per Serving):**

Calories 140  Fat 3.6 g  Carbs 5 g  Sugar 2 g  Protein 22 g  Cholesterol 54 mg

# Easy Spinach Muffins

**Time:** 25 minutes

**Serve:** 12

**Ingredients:**

- 10 eggs
- 2 cups spinach, chopped
- 1/4 tsp garlic powder
- 1/4 tsp onion powder
- 1/2 tsp dried basil
- 1 1/2 cups parmesan cheese, grated
- Salt

**Directions:**

1. Preheat the oven to 400 F. Grease muffin tin and set aside.
2. In a large bowl, whisk eggs with basil, garlic powder, onion powder, and salt.
3. Add cheese and spinach and stir well.
4. Pour egg mixture into the prepared muffin tin and bake 15 minutes.
5. Serve and enjoy.

**Nutritional Value (Amount per Serving):**

Calories 110  Fat 7 g  Carbs 1 g  Sugar 0.3 g  Protein 9 g  Cholesterol 165 mg

# Healthy Cauliflower Grits

**Time:** 2 hours 10 minutes

**Serve:** 8

**Ingredients:**

- 6 cups cauliflower rice
- 1/4 tsp garlic powder
- 1 cup cream cheese
- 1/2 cup vegetable stock
- 1/4 tsp onion powder
- 1/2 tsp pepper
- 1 tsp salt

**Directions:**

1. Add all ingredients into the slow cooker and stir well combine.
2. Cover and cook on low for 2 hours.
3. Stir and serve.

**Nutritional Value (Amount per Serving):**

Calories 126  Fat 10 g  Carbs 5 g  Sugar 2 g  Protein 4 g  Cholesterol 31 mg

# Spinach Tomato Frittata

**Time:** 30 minutes

**Serve:** 8

**Ingredients:**

- 12 eggs
- 2 cups baby spinach, shredded
- 1/4 cup sun-dried tomatoes, sliced
- 1/2 tsp dried basil
- 1/4 cup parmesan cheese, grated
- Pepper
- Salt

**Directions:**

1. Preheat the oven to 425 F. Grease oven-safe pan and set aside.
2. In a large bowl, whisk eggs with pepper and salt. Add remaining ingredients and stir to combine.
3. Pour egg mixture into the prepared pan and bake for 20 minutes.
4. Slice and serve.

**Nutritional Value (Amount per Serving):**

Calories 116  Fat 7 g  Carbs 1 g  Sugar 1 g  Protein 10 g  Cholesterol 250 mg

# Tofu Scramble

**Time:** 17 minutes

**Serve:** 2

**Ingredients:**

- 1/2 block firm tofu, crumbled
- 1 cup spinach
- 1/4 cup zucchini, chopped
- 1 tbsp olive oil
- 1 tomato, chopped
- 1/4 tsp ground cumin
- 1 tbsp turmeric
- 1 tbsp coriander, chopped
- 1 tbsp chives, chopped
- Pepper
- Salt

**Directions:**

1. Heat oil in a pan over medium heat.
2. Add tomato, zucchini, and spinach and sauté for 2 minutes.
3. Add tofu, turmeric, cumin, pepper, and salt, and sauté for 5 minutes.
4. Garnish with chives and coriander.
5. Serve and enjoy.

**Nutritional Value (Amount per Serving):**

Calories 102  Fat 8 g  Carbs 5 g  Sugar 2 g  Protein 3 g  Cholesterol 0 mg

# Shrimp & Zucchini

**Time:** 30 minutes

**Serve:** 4

**Ingredients:**

- 1 lb shrimp, peeled and deveined
- 1 zucchini, chopped
- 1 summer squash, chopped
- 2 tbsp olive oil
- 1/2 small onion, chopped
- 1/2 tsp paprika
- 1/2 tsp garlic powder
- 1/2 tsp onion powder
- Pepper
- Salt

**Directions:**

1. In a bowl, mix together paprika, garlic powder, onion powder, pepper, and salt. Add shrimp and toss well.
2. Heat 1 tablespoon of oil in a pan over medium heat,
3. Add shrimp and cook for 2 minutes on each side or until shrimp turns to pink.
4. Transfer shrimp on a plate.
5. Add remaining oil in a pan.
6. Add onion, summer squash, and zucchini and cook for 6-8 minutes or until vegetables are softened.
7. Return shrimp to the pan and cook for 1 minute.
8. Serve and enjoy.

**Nutritional Value (Amount per Serving):**

Calories 215  Fat 9 g  Carbs 6 g  Sugar 2 g  Protein 27 g  Cholesterol 239 mg

# Baked Dijon Salmon

**Time:** 30 minutes

**Serve:** 5

**Ingredients:**

- 1 1/2 lbs salmon
- 1/4 cup Dijon mustard
- 1/4 cup fresh parsley, chopped
- 1 tbsp garlic, chopped
- 1 tbsp olive oil
- 1 tbsp fresh lemon juice
- Pepper
- Salt

**Directions:**

1. Preheat the oven to 375 F. Line baking sheet with parchment paper.
2. Arrange salmon fillets on a prepared baking sheet.
3. In a small bowl, mix together garlic, oil, lemon juice, Dijon mustard, parsley, pepper, and salt.
4. Brush salmon top with garlic mixture.
5. Bake for 18-20 minutes.
6. Serve and enjoy.

**Nutritional Value (Amount per Serving):**

Calories 217  Fat 11 g  Carbs 2 g  Sugar 0.2 g  Protein 27 g  Cholesterol 60 mg

# Cauliflower Spinach Rice

**Time:** 15 minutes

**Serve:** 4

**Ingredients:**

- 5 oz baby spinach
- 4 cups cauliflower rice
- 1 tsp garlic, minced
- 3 tbsp olive oil
- 1 fresh lime juice
- 1/4 cup vegetable broth
- 1/4 tsp chili powder
- Pepper
- Salt

**Directions:**

1. Heat olive oil in a pan over medium heat.
2. Add garlic and sauté for 30 seconds. Add cauliflower rice, chili powder, pepper, and salt and cook for 2 minutes.
3. Add broth and lime juice and stir well.
4. Add spinach and stir until spinach is wilted.
5. Serve and enjoy.

**Nutritional Value (Amount per Serving):**

Calories 147  Fat 11 g  Carbs 9 g  Sugar 4 g  Protein 5 g  Cholesterol 23 mg

# Cauliflower Broccoli Mash

**Time:** 22 minutes

**Serve:** 3

**Ingredients:**

- 1 lb cauliflower, cut into florets
- 2 cups broccoli, chopped
- 1 tsp garlic, minced
- 1 tsp dried rosemary
- 1/4 cup olive oil
- Salt

**Directions:**

1. Add broccoli and cauliflower into the instant pot.
2. Pour enough water into the instant pot to cover broccoli and cauliflower.
3. Seal pot and cook on high pressure for 12 minutes.
4. Once done, allow to release pressure naturally. Remove lid.
5. Drain broccoli and cauliflower and clean the instant pot.
6. Add oil into the instant pot and set the pot on sauté mode.
7. Add broccoli, cauliflower, rosemary, garlic, and salt and cook for 10 minutes.
8. Mash the broccoli and cauliflower mixture using a masher until smooth.
9. Serve and enjoy.

**Nutritional Value (Amount per Serving):**

Calories 205  Fat 17 g  Carbs 12 g  Sugar 5 g  Protein 5 g  Cholesterol 0 mg

# Italian Chicken Soup

**Time:** 35 minutes

**Serve:** 6

**Ingredients:**

- 1 lb chicken breasts, boneless and cut into chunks
- 1 1/2 cups salsa
- 1 tsp Italian seasoning
- 2 tbsp fresh parsley, chopped
- 3 cups chicken stock
- 8 oz cream cheese
- Pepper
- Salt

**Directions:**

1. Add all ingredients except cream cheese and parsley into the instant pot and stir well.
2. Seal pot and cook on high pressure for 25 minutes.
3. Release pressure using quick release. Remove lid.
4. Remove chicken from pot and shred using a fork.
5. Return shredded chicken to the instant pot.
6. Add cream cheese and stir well and cook on sauté mode until cheese is melted.
7. Serve and enjoy.

**Nutritional Value (Amount per Serving):**

Calories 300  Fat 19 g  Carbs 5 g  Sugar 2 g  Protein 26 g  Cholesterol 109 mg

# Tasty Tomatoes Soup

**Time:** 15 minutes

**Serve:** 2

**Ingredients:**

- 14 oz can fire-roasted tomatoes
- 1/2 tsp dried basil
- 1/2 cup heavy cream
- 1/2 cup parmesan cheese, grated
- 1 cup cheddar cheese, grated
- 1 1/2 cups vegetable stock
- 1/4 cup zucchini, grated
- 1/2 tsp dried oregano
- Pepper
- Salt

**Directions:**

1. Add tomatoes, stock, zucchini, oregano, basil, pepper, and salt into the instant pot and stir well.
2. Seal pot and cook on high pressure for 5 minutes.
3. Release pressure using quick release. Remove lid.
4. Set pot on sauté mode. Add heavy cream, parmesan cheese, and cheddar cheese and stir well and cook until cheese is melted.
5. Serve and enjoy.

**Nutritional Value (Amount per Serving):**

Calories 460  Fat 35 g  Carbs 13 g  Sugar 6 g  Protein 24 g  Cholesterol 117 mg

# Cauliflower Spinach Soup

**Time:** 20 minutes

**Serve:** 2

**Ingredients:**

- 3 cups spinach, chopped
- 1 cup cauliflower, chopped
- 2 tbsp olive oil
- 3 cups vegetable broth
- 1/2 cup heavy cream
- 1 tsp garlic powder
- Pepper
- Salt

**Directions:**

1. Add all ingredients except cream into the instant pot and stir well.
2. Seal pot and cook on high pressure for 10 minutes.
3. Release pressure using quick release. Remove lid.
4. Stir in cream and blend soup using a blender until smooth.
5. Serve and enjoy.

**Nutritional Value (Amount per Serving):**

Calories 310  Fat 27 g  Carbs 7 g  Sugar 3 g  Protein 10 g  Cholesterol 41 mg

# Delicious Chicken Salad

**Time:** 15 minutes

**Serve:** 4

**Ingredients:**

- 1 1/2 cups chicken breast, skinless, boneless, and cooked
- 2 tbsp onion, diced
- 1/4 cup olives, diced
- 1/4 cup roasted red peppers, diced
- 1/4 cup cucumbers, diced
- 1/4 cup celery, diced
- 1/4 cup feta cheese, crumbled
- 1/2 tsp onion powder
- 1/2 tbsp fresh lemon juice
- 1 tbsp fresh parsley, chopped
- 1 tbsp fresh dill, chopped
- 2 1/2 tbsp mayonnaise
- 1/4 cup Greek yogurt
- 1/4 tsp pepper
- 1/2 tsp salt

**Directions:**

1. In a bowl, mix together yogurt, onion powder, lemon juice, parsley, dill, mayonnaise, pepper, and salt.
2. Add chicken, onion, olives, red peppers, cucumbers, and feta cheese and stir well.
3. Serve and enjoy.

**Nutritional Value (Amount per Serving):**

Calories 172  Fat 7.9 g  Carbs 6.7 g  Sugar 3.1 g  Protein 18.1 g  Cholesterol 52 mg

# Baked Pesto Salmon

**Time:** 30 minutes

**Serve:** 5

**Ingredients:**

- 1 3/4 lbs salmon fillet
- 1/3 cup basil pesto
- 1/4 cup sun-dried tomatoes, drained
- 1/4 cup olives, pitted and chopped
- 1 tbsp fresh dill, chopped
- 1/4 cup capers
- 1/3 cup artichoke hearts
- 1 tsp paprika
- 1/4 tsp salt

**Directions:**

1. Preheat the oven to 400 F. Line baking sheet with parchment paper.
2. Arrange salmon fillet on a prepared baking sheet and season with paprika and salt.
3. Add remaining ingredients on top of salmon and spread evenly.
4. Bake for 20 minutes.
5. Serve and enjoy.

**Nutritional Value (Amount per Serving):**

Calories 228  Fat 10.7 g  Carbs 2.7 g  Sugar 0.3 g  Protein 31.6 g  Cholesterol 70 mg

# Easy Shrimp Salad

**Time:** 15 minutes

**Serve:** 6

**Ingredients:**

- 2 lbs shrimp, cooked
- 1/4 cup onion, minced
- 1/4 cup fresh dill, chopped
- 1/3 cup fresh chives, chopped
- 1/2 cup fresh celery, chopped
- 1/4 tsp cayenne pepper
- 1 tbsp fresh lemon juice
- 1 tbsp olive oil
- 1/4 cup mayonnaise
- 1/4 tsp pepper
- 1/4 tsp salt

**Directions:**

1. In a large bowl, add all ingredients except shrimp and mix well.
2. Add shrimp and toss well.
3. Serve and enjoy.

**Nutritional Value (Amount per Serving):**

Calories 248  Fat 8.3 g  Carbs 6.7 g  Sugar 1.1 g  Protein 35.2 g  Cholesterol 321 mg

# Simple Haddock Salad

**Time:** 15 minutes

**Serve:** 6

**Ingredients:**

- 1 lb haddock, cooked
- 1 tbsp green onion, chopped
- 1 tbsp olive oil
- 1 tsp garlic, minced
- Pepper
- Salt

**Directions:**

1. Cut cooked haddock into the bite-size pieces and place on a plate.
2. Drizzle with oil and season with pepper and salt.
3. Sprinkle garlic and green onion over haddock.
4. Serve and enjoy.

**Nutritional Value (Amount per Serving):**

Calories 106  Fat 3 g  Carbs 0.2 g  Sugar 0 g  Protein 18.4 g  Cholesterol 56 mg

# Baked White Fish Fillet

**Time:** 40 minutes

**Serve:** 1

**Ingredients:**

- 8 oz frozen white fish fillet
- 1 tbsp roasted red bell pepper, diced
- 1/2 tsp Italian seasoning
- 1 tbsp fresh parsley, chopped
- 1 1/2 tbsp olive oil
- 1 tbsp lemon juice

**Directions:**

1. Preheat the oven to 400 F. Line baking sheet with foil.
2. Place a fish fillet on a baking sheet.
3. Drizzle oil and lemon juice over fish. Season with Italian seasoning.
4. Top with roasted bell pepper and parsley and bake for 30 minutes.
5. Serve and enjoy.

**Nutritional Value (Amount per Serving):**

Calories 383  Fat 22.5 g  Carbs 0.8 g  Sugar 0.6 g  Protein 46.5 g  Cholesterol 2 mg

## Air Fry Salmon

**Time:** 25 minutes

**Serve:** 4

**Ingredients:**

- 1 lbs salmon, cut into 4 pieces
- 1 tbsp olive oil
- 1/2 tbsp dried rosemary
- 1/4 tsp dried basil
- 1 tbsp dried chives
- Pepper
- Salt

**Directions:**

1. Place salmon pieces skin side down into the air fryer basket.
2. In a small bowl, mix together olive oil, basil, chives, and rosemary.
3. Brush salmon with oil mixture and air fry at 400 F for 15 minutes.
4. Serve and enjoy.

**Nutritional Value (Amount per Serving):**

Calories 182  Fat 10.6 g  Carbs 0.3 g  Sugar 0 g  Protein 22 g  Cholesterol 50 mg

# Baked Salmon Patties

**Time:** 30 minutes

**Serve:** 4

**Ingredients:**

- 2 eggs, lightly beaten
- 14 oz can salmon, drained and flaked with a fork
- 1 tbsp garlic, minced
- 1/4 cup almond flour
- 1/2 cup fresh parsley, chopped
- 1 tsp Dijon mustard
- 1/4 tsp pepper
- 1/2 tsp kosher salt

**Directions:**

1. Preheat the oven to 400 F. Line a baking sheet with parchment paper and set aside.
2. Add all ingredients into the bowl and mix until well combined.
3. Make small patties from mixture and place on a prepared baking sheet.
4. Bake patties for 10 minutes.
5. Turn patties and bake for 10 minutes more.
6. Serve and enjoy.

**Nutritional Value (Amount per Serving):**

Calories 216  Fat 11.8 g  Carbs 3 g  Sugar 0.5 g  Protein 24.3 g  Cholesterol 136 mg

# FUELING RECIPES
## Chocolate Bars

**Time:** 20 minutes

**Serve:** 16

**Ingredients:**

- 15 oz cream cheese, softened
- 15 oz unsweetened dark chocolate
- 1 tsp vanilla
- 10 drops liquid stevia

**Directions:**

1. Grease 8-inch square dish and set aside.
2. Melt chocolate in a saucepan over low heat.
3. Add stevia and vanilla and stir well.
4. Remove pan from heat and set aside.
5. Add cream cheese into the blender and blend until smooth.
6. Add melted chocolate mixture into the cream cheese and blend until just combined.
7. Transfer mixture into the prepared dish and spread evenly and place in the refrigerator until firm.
8. Slice and serve.

**Nutritional Value (Amount per Serving):**

Calories 230  Fat 24 g  Carbs 7.5 g  Sugar 0.1 g  Protein 6 g  Cholesterol 29 mg

# Blueberry Muffins

**Time:** 35 minutes

**Serve:** 12

**Ingredients:**

- 2 eggs
- 1/2 cup fresh blueberries
- 1 cup heavy cream
- 2 cups almond flour
- 1/4 tsp lemon zest
- 1/2 tsp lemon extract
- 1 tsp baking powder
- 5 drops stevia
- 1/4 cup butter, melted

**Directions:**

1. Preheat the oven to 350 F. Line muffin tin with cupcake liners and set aside.
2. Add eggs into the bowl and whisk until mix.
3. Add remaining ingredients and mix to combine.
4. Pour mixture into the prepared muffin tin and bake for 25 minutes.
5. Serve and enjoy.

**Nutritional Value (Amount per Serving):**

Calories 190  Fat 17 g  Carbs 5 g  Sugar 1 g  Protein 5 g  Cholesterol 55 mg

# Chia Pudding

**Time:** 20 minutes

**Serve:** 2

**Ingredients:**

- 4 tbsp chia seeds
- 1 cup unsweetened coconut milk
- 1/2 cup raspberries

**Directions:**

1. Add raspberry and coconut milk into a blender and blend until smooth.
2. Pour mixture into the glass jar.
3. Add chia seeds in a jar and stir well.
4. Seal the jar with a lid and shake well and place in the refrigerator for 3 hours.
5. Serve chilled and enjoy.

**Nutritional Value (Amount per Serving):**

Calories 360  Fat 33 g  Carbs 13 g  Sugar 5 g  Protein 6 g  Cholesterol 0 mg

# Avocado Pudding

**Time:** 20 minutes

**Serve:** 8

**Ingredients:**

- 2 ripe avocados, peeled, pitted and cut into pieces
- 1 tbsp fresh lime juice
- 14 oz can coconut milk
- 2 tsp liquid stevia
- 2 tsp vanilla

**Directions:**

1. Add all ingredients into the blender and blend until smooth.
2. Serve immediately and enjoy.

**Nutritional Value (Amount per Serving):**

Calories 317  Fat 30 g  Carbs 9 g  Sugar 0.5 g  Protein 3 g  Cholesterol 0 mg

# Peanut Butter Coconut Popsicle

**Time:** 15 minutes

**Serve:** 12

**Ingredients:**

- 1/2 cup peanut butter
- 1 tsp liquid stevia
- 2 cans unsweetened coconut milk

**Directions:**

1. Add all ingredients into the blender and blend until smooth.
2. Pour mixture into the Popsicle molds and place in the freezer for 4 hours or until set.
3. Serve and enjoy.

**Nutritional Value (Amount per Serving):**

Calories 155  Fat 15 g  Carbs 4 g  Sugar 2 g  Protein 3 g  Cholesterol 0 mg

# Delicious Brownie Bites

**Time:** 20 minutes

**Serve:** 13

**Ingredients:**

- 1/4 cup unsweetened chocolate chips
- 1/4 cup unsweetened cocoa powder
- 1 cup pecans, chopped
- 1/2 cup almond butter
- 1/2 tsp vanilla
- 1/4 cup monk fruit sweetener
- 1/8 tsp pink salt

**Directions:**

1. Add pecans, sweetener, vanilla, almond butter, cocoa powder, and salt into the food processor and process until well combined.
2. Transfer brownie mixture into the large bowl. Add chocolate chips and fold well.
3. Make small round shape balls from brownie mixture and place onto a baking tray.
4. Place in the freezer for 20 minutes.
5. Serve and enjoy.

**Nutritional Value (Amount per Serving):**

Calories 108  Fat 9 g  Carbs 4 g  Sugar 1 g  Protein 2 g  Cholesterol 0 mg

# Pumpkin Balls

**Time:** 15 minutes

**Serve:** 18

**Ingredients:**

- 1 cup almond butter
- 5 drops liquid stevia
- 2 tbsp coconut flour
- 2 tbsp pumpkin puree
- 1 tsp pumpkin pie spice

**Directions:**

1. In a large bowl, mix together pumpkin puree and almond butter until well combined.
2. Add liquid stevia, pumpkin pie spice, and coconut flour and mix well.
3. Make small balls from mixture and place onto a baking tray.
4. Place in the freezer for 1 hour.
5. Serve and enjoy.

**Nutritional Value (Amount per Serving):**

Calories 96  Fat 8 g  Carbs 4 g  Sugar 1 g  Protein 2 g  Cholesterol 0 mg

# Smooth Peanut Butter Cream

**Time:** 10 minutes

**Serve:** 8

**Ingredients:**

- 1/4 cup peanut butter
- 4 overripe bananas, chopped
- 1/3 cup cocoa powder
- 1/4 tsp vanilla extract
- 1/8 tsp salt

**Directions:**

1. Add all ingredients into the blender and blend until smooth.
2. Serve immediately and enjoy.

**Nutritional Value (Amount per Serving):**

Calories 101  Fat 5 g  Carbs 14 g  Sugar 7 g  Protein 3 g  Cholesterol 0 mg

# Vanilla Avocado Popsicles

**Time:** 20 minutes

**Serve:** 6

**Ingredients:**

- 2 avocadoes
- 1 tsp vanilla
- 1 cup almond milk
- 1 tsp liquid stevia
- 1/2 cup unsweetened cocoa powder

**Directions:**

1. Add all ingredients into the blender and blend until smooth.
2. Pour blended mixture into the Popsicle molds and place in the freezer until set.
3. Serve and enjoy.

**Nutritional Value (Amount per Serving):**

Calories 130  Fat 12 g  Carbs 7 g  Sugar 1 g  Protein 3 g  Cholesterol 0 mg

# Chocolate Popsicle

**Time:** 20 minutes

**Serve:** 6

**Ingredients:**

- 4 oz unsweetened chocolate, chopped
- 6 drops liquid stevia
- 1 1/2 cups heavy cream

**Directions:**

1. Add heavy cream into the microwave-safe bowl and microwave until just begins the boiling.
2. Add chocolate into the heavy cream and set aside for 5 minutes.
3. Add liquid stevia into the heavy cream mixture and stir until chocolate is melted.
4. Pour mixture into the Popsicle molds and place in freezer for 4 hours or until set.
5. Serve and enjoy.

**Nutritional Value (Amount per Serving):**

Calories 198  Fat 21 g  Carbs 6 g  Sugar 0.2 g  Protein 3 g  Cholesterol 41 mg

# Raspberry Ice Cream

**Time:** 10 minutes

**Serve:** 2

**Ingredients:**

- 1 cup frozen raspberries
- 1/2 cup heavy cream
- 1/8 tsp stevia powder

**Directions:**

1. Add all ingredients into the blender and blend until smooth.
2. Serve immediately and enjoy.

**Nutritional Value (Amount per Serving):**

Calories 144  Fat 11 g  Carbs 10 g  Sugar 4 g  Protein 2 g  Cholesterol 41 mg

# Chocolate Frosty

**Time:** 20 minutes

**Serve:** 4

**Ingredients:**

- 2 tbsp unsweetened cocoa powder
- 1 cup heavy whipping cream
- 1 tbsp almond butter
- 5 drops liquid stevia
- 1 tsp vanilla

**Directions:**

1. Add cream into the medium bowl and beat using the hand mixer for 5 minutes.
2. Add remaining ingredients and blend until thick cream form.
3. Pour in serving bowls and place them in the freezer for 30 minutes.
4. Serve and enjoy.

**Nutritional Value (Amount per Serving):**

Calories 137  Fat 13 g  Carbs 3 g  Sugar 0.5 g  Protein 2 g  Cholesterol 41 mg

# Chocolate Almond Butter Brownie

**Time:** 26 minutes

**Serve:** 4

**Ingredients:**

- 1 cup bananas, overripe
- 1/2 cup almond butter, melted
- 1 scoop protein powder
- 2 tbsp unsweetened cocoa powder

**Directions:**

1. Preheat the air fryer to 325 F. Grease air fryer baking pan and set aside.
2. Add all ingredients into the blender and blend until smooth.
3. Pour batter into the prepared pan and place in the air fryer basket and cook for 16 minutes.
4. Serve and enjoy.

**Nutritional Value (Amount per Serving):**

Calories 82  Fat 2 g  Carbs 11 g  Sugar 5 g  Protein 7 g  Cholesterol 16 mg

# Peanut Butter Fudge

**Time:** 20 minutes

**Serve:** 20

**Ingredients:**

- 1/4 cup almonds, toasted and chopped
- 12 oz smooth peanut butter
- 15 drops liquid stevia
- 3 tbsp coconut oil
- 4 tbsp coconut cream
- Pinch of salt

**Directions:**

1. Line baking tray with parchment paper.
2. Melt coconut oil in a saucepan over low heat. Add peanut butter, coconut cream, stevia, and salt in a saucepan. Stir well.
3. Pour fudge mixture into the prepared baking tray and sprinkle chopped almonds on top.
4. Place the tray in the refrigerator for 1 hour or until set.
5. Slice and serve.

**Nutritional Value (Amount per Serving):**

Calories 131  Fat 12 g  Carbs 4 g  Sugar 2 g  Protein 5 g  Cholesterol 0 mg

# Almond Butter Fudge

**Time:** 10 minutes

**Serve:** 18

**Ingredients:**

- 3/4 cup creamy almond butter
- 1 1/2 cups unsweetened chocolate chips

**Directions:**

1. Line 8*4-inch pan with parchment paper and set aside.
2. Add chocolate chips and almond butter into the double boiler and cook over medium heat until the chocolate-butter mixture is melted. Stir well.
3. Pour mixture into the prepared pan and place in the freezer until set.
4. Slice and serve.

**Nutritional Value (Amount per Serving):**

Calories 197  Fat 16 g  Carbs 7 g  Sugar 1 g  Protein 4 g  Cholesterol 0 mg

# Mocha Mousse

**Time:** 20 minutes

**Serve:** 8

**Ingredients:**

- 1/2 cup coffee strong brewed, cooled
- 2 cups heavy whipping cream
- 6 oz unsweetened chocolate, chopped
- 1 tsp coffee extract

**Directions:**

1. In a large bowl, whip heavy cream and set aside.
2. Melt chocolate in a microwave-safe bowl.
3. Add coffee and coffee extract in melted chocolate and stir well.
4. Pour chocolate mixture into the whipped cream and stir until just combined.
5. Place in refrigerator for 30 minutes.
6. Serve and enjoy.

**Nutritional Value (Amount per Serving):**

Calories 211  Fat 22 g  Carbs 7 g  Sugar 0.2 g  Protein 3 g  Cholesterol 41 mg

# Pumpkin Mousse

**Time:** 20 minutes

**Serve:** 12

**Ingredients:**

- 2 tsp pumpkin pie spice
- 1 tsp liquid stevia
- 2 cups heavy cream
- 15 oz can pumpkin puree
- 15 oz cream cheese
- 1 tsp vanilla
- Pinch of salt

**Directions:**

1. In a large bowl, blend together pumpkin and cream cheese until smooth.
2. Add remaining ingredients and beat until fluffy.
3. Pipe into the serving glasses and place in the refrigerator for 1 hour.
4. Serve and enjoy.

**Nutritional Value (Amount per Serving):**

Calories 209  Fat 19 g  Carbs 5 g  Sugar 1 g  Protein 3 g  Cholesterol 66 mg

# Chocolate Mousse

**Time:** 10 minutes

**Serve:** 4

**Ingredients:**

- 1/2 cup unsweetened cocoa powder
- 1 1/4 cup heavy cream
- 5 drop stevia
- 4 oz cream cheese
- 1/2 tsp vanilla

**Directions:**

1. Add all ingredients to the blender and blend until smooth and.
2. Pipe mixture into the serving glasses and place them in the refrigerator for 1 hour.
3. Serve chilled and enjoy.

**Nutritional Value (Amount per Serving):**

Calories 254  Fat 25 g  Carbs 7 g  Sugar 0.4 g  Protein 5 g  Cholesterol 83 mg

# Pound Cake

**Time:** 65 minutes

**Serve:** 10

**Ingredients:**

- 4 eggs
- 1/4 cup cream cheese
- 1/4 cup butter
- 1 tsp baking powder
- 1 tbsp coconut flour
- 1 cup almond flour
- 1/2 cup sour cream
- 1 tsp vanilla
- 1 cup monk fruit sweetener

**Directions:**

1. Preheat the oven to 350 F. Grease 9-inch cake pan and set aside.
2. In a large bowl, mix together almond flour, baking powder, and coconut flour.
3. In a separate bowl, add cream cheese and butter and microwave for 30 seconds. Stir well and microwave for 30 seconds more.
4. Stir in sour cream, vanilla, and sweetener. Stir well.
5. Pour cream cheese mixture into the almond flour mixture and stir until just combined.
6. Add eggs in batter one by one and stir until well combined.
7. Pour batter into the prepared cake pan and bake for 55 minutes.
8. Remove cake from the oven and let it cool completely.
9. Slice and serve.

**Nutritional Value (Amount per Serving):**

Calories 211  Fat 17 g  Carbs 8 g  Sugar 5 g  Protein 3 g  Cholesterol 89 mg

# Almond Butter Cookies

**Time:** 28 minutes

**Serve:** 7

**Ingredients:**

- 6 oz almond butter
- 1/3 cup pumpkin puree
- 1/4 tsp pumpkin pie spice
- 1 tsp liquid stevia

**Directions:**

1. Preheat the oven to 350 F. Line baking sheet with parchment paper and set aside.
2. Add all ingredients into the food processor and process until just combined.
3. Drop spoonfuls of mixture onto the prepared baking sheet.
4. Bake for 18 minutes.
5. Let the cookies cool completely.
6. Serve and enjoy.

**Nutritional Value (Amount per Serving):**

Calories 88  Fat 7 g  Carbs 3 g  Sugar 1 g  Protein 3 g  Cholesterol 0 mg